The Vibrant Keto Vegetarian Cooking Book

A Set of Super Easy and Quick Recipes Perfect for Every Occasion

Tia Graham

Table of contents

Orange Juice Smoothie

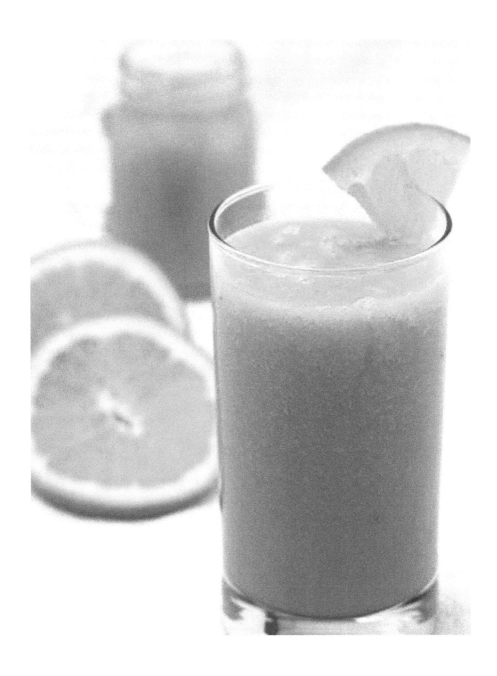

Preparation Time: 5 mins Servings: 2

Ingredients:

¼ c. frozen orange juice concentrate

¾ c. fat-free milk

1 c. fat-free vanilla frozen yogurt

Directions:

1.   Add the ingredients to a blender and pulse until they're smooth.

2.   Pour them into frosted glasses and serve.

Nutrition: Calories: 180, Fat:0 g, Carbs:38 g, Protein:7 g, Sugars:20 g, Sodium:5 mg

Chocolate Aquafaba Mousse

Preparation Time: 20 mins Servings: 4-6

Ingredients:

1 tsp. pure vanilla extract

15 oz. unsalted chickpeas Fresh raspberries

¼ tsp. tartar cream

6 oz. dairy-free dark chocolate 2 tbsps. coconut sugar

¼ tsp. sea salt

Directions

1.   Chop dark chocolate into coarse bits and place the chocolate into a glass bowl over boiling water on the stovetop or in a double boiler.

2.   Melt the chocolate gently, stirring until completely melted.

3.   Remove the melted chocolate from the heat and pour the chocolate into a large bowl.

4.   Drain the chickpeas, reserving the brine (aquafaba), and store the chickpeas for another recipe like hummus.

5.   Add in the aquafaba along with cream of tartar.

6.   Mix on high speed using an electric hand mixer for 7-10 minutes, or until soft peaks begin to form.

7.   Add in the salt, vanilla extract, and coconut sugar and beat the mixture until well mixed.

8.   Add half of the melted chocolate to the whipped aquafaba and fold it in until incorporated.

9.   Fold in the remaining aquafaba until smooth and well combined to form the mousse.

10.   Gently spoon the chocolate mousse into glasses, ramekins or small mason jars.

11.   Cover with cling film and chill for at least 3 hours.

12.   Sprinkle he mousse with raspberries and serve.

Nutrition: Calories: 280, Fat:13.8 g, Carbs:34.7 g, Protein:3.9 g, Sugars:22 g, Sodium:242 mg

Minted Peas Feta Rice

Preparation Time: 15 mins Servings: 2

Ingredients:

1 ¼ c. vegetable broth

¾ c. brown rice

¼ c. finely crumbled feta cheese

¾ c. sliced scallions

1 ½ c. frozen peas

Freshly ground pepper

¼ c. sliced fresh mint

Directions:

1.   Boil broth in a saucepan over medium heat.

2.   Add rice and bring it to a simmer. Cook for 4 minutes.

3.   Stir in peas and cook for 6 minutes.

4.   Turn off the heat then add feta, mint, scallions, and pepper.

5.   Serve warm.

Nutrition: Calories: 28.1, Fat:18.2 g, Carbs:10.3 g, Protein:8.8 g, Sugars:2.2 g, Sodium:216 mg

Hearty Baby Carrots

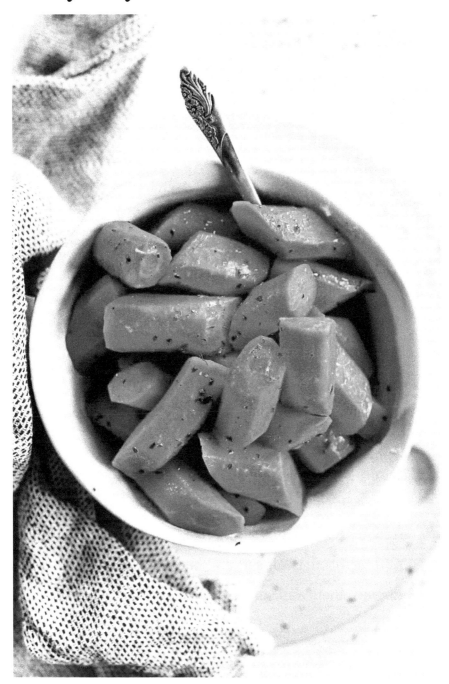

Preparation Time: 5 mins Servings: 4

Ingredients:

1 tbsp. chopped fresh mint

1 c. water

Sea flavored vinegar

1 lb. baby carrots

1 tbsp. clarified ghee

Directions:

1. Place a steamer rack on top of your pot and add the carrots

2. Add water

3. Lock up the lid and cook at HIGH pressure for 2 minutes

4. Do a quick release

5. Pass the carrots through a strainer and drain them

6. Wipe the insert clean

7. Return the insert to the pot and set the pot to Sauté mode

8. Add clarified butter and allow it to melt

9. Add mint and sauté for 30 seconds

10. Add carrots to the insert and sauté well

11. Remove them and sprinkle with bit of flavored vinegar on top

12. Enjoy!

Nutrition: Calories: 131, Fat:10 g, Carbs:11 g, Protein:1 g, Sugars:5 g, Sodium:190 mg

Sensitive Steamed Artichokes

Preparation Time: 5 mins Servings: 4

Ingredients:

1   halved lemon

¼ tsp. paprika

2   tbsps. Homemade Whole

30 mayo 2 medium artichokes

1 tsp. Dijon mustard

Directions:

1.   Wash the artichokes and remove the damaged outer leaves

2.   Trim the spines and cut off upper edge

3.   Wipe the cur edges with lemon half

4.   Slice the stem and peel the stem

5.   Chop it up and keep them on the side

6.   Add a cup of water to the pot and place a steamer basket inside

7.   Transfer the artichokes to the steamer basket and a squeeze of lemon

8.   Lock up the lid and cook on HIGH pressure for 10 minutes

9.   Release the pressure naturally

10.   Enjoy

Nutrition: Calories: 77, Fat:5 g, Carbs:0 g, Protein:2 g, Sugars:1.3 g, Sodium:121 mg

Rhubarb and Strawberry Compote

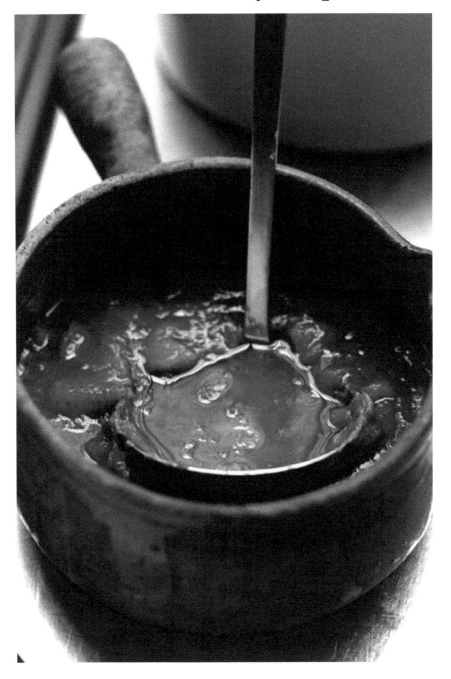

Preparation Time: 10 mins Servings: 4

Ingredients:

3 tbsps. Date paste

½ c. water Fresh mint

2 lbs. rhubarb

1   lb. strawberries

Directions:

1.   Peel the rhubarb using a paring knife and chop it up ½ inch pieces

2.   Add the chopped up rhubarb to your pot alongside water

3.   Lock up the lid and cook on HIGH pressure for 10 minutes

4.   Stem and quarter your strawberries and keep them on the side

5.   Add the strawberries and date paste, give it a nice stir

6.   Lock up the lid and cook on HIGH pressure for 20 minutes

7.   Release the pressure naturally and enjoy the compote!

Nutrition: Calories: 41.1, Fat:2.1 g, Carbs:5.5 g, Protein:1.4 g, Sugars:12 g, Sodium:2.4 mg

Zucchini Cakes

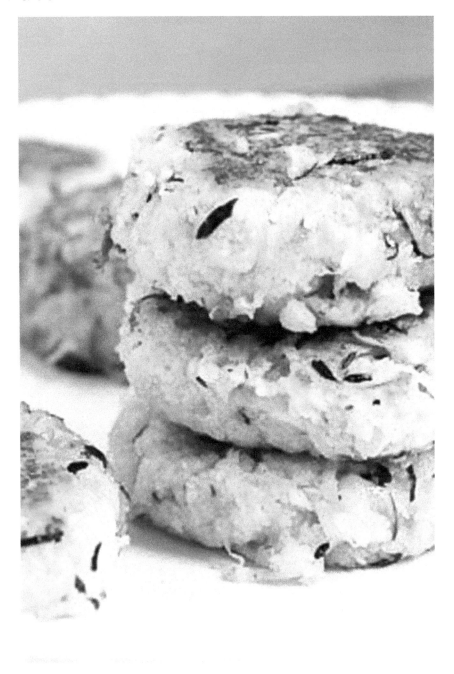

Preparation Time: 10 mins Servings: 4

Ingredients:

Freshly ground black pepper

1 finely diced red onion

2   tsps. Salt

1 egg white

Homemade horseradish sauce

1 shredded medium zucchini

¾ c. salt-free breadcrumbs

Directions:

1.   Preheat oven to 400°F. Spray a baking sheet lightly with oil and set aside.

2.   Press shredded zucchini gently between paper towels to remove excess liquid.

3.   In a large bowl, combine zucchini, onion, egg white, breadcrumbs, seasoning, and black pepper. Mix well.

4.   Shape mixture into patties and place on the prepared baking sheet.

5.   Place baking sheet on middle rack in oven and bake for 10 minutes. Gently flip patties and return to oven to bake for another 10 minutes.

6.   Remove from oven and serve immediately.

Nutrition: Calories: 94, Fat:1 g, Carbs:19 g, Protein:4 g, Sugars:31 g, Sodium:161 mg

Fresh Fruit Smoothie

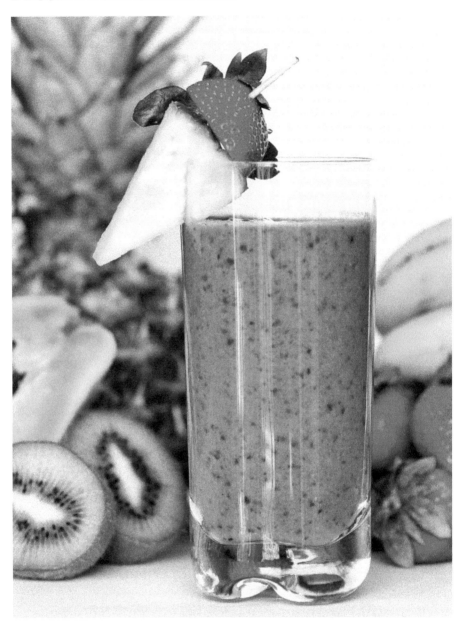

Preparation Time: 5 mins Servings: 4

Ingredients:

1 tbsp. honey

½ c. cantaloupe 1 c. water

1   c. fresh strawberries

1 c. fresh pineapple

2   orange juice

Directions:

1.   Remove the rind from the melon and pineapple. Cut them into chunks and remove the stems from the strawberries.

2.   Put everything in a blender and serve.

Nutrition: Calories: 72, Fat:1 g, Carbs:17 g, Protein:1 g, Sugars:1 g, Sodium:42 mg

Popovers

Preparation Time: 5 mins Servings: 6

Ingredients:

4 egg whites

1   c. All-purpose flour

1 c. fat-free milk

¼ tsp. salt

Directions:

1.   Preheat your oven to 425 0F.

2.   Coat a six cup metal or glass muffin mold with cooking spray and heat the mold in the oven for two minutes.

3.   In a bowl, add the flour, milk, salt, and egg whites. Use a mixer to beat until it's smooth.

4.   Fill the heated molds two-thirds of the way full.

5.   Bake until the muffins are golden brown and puffy, around half an hour. Serve.

Nutrition: Calories: 101, Fat:0 g, Carbs:18 g, Protein:6 g, Sugars:2 g, Sodium:125 mg

Broccoli, Garlic, and Rigatoni

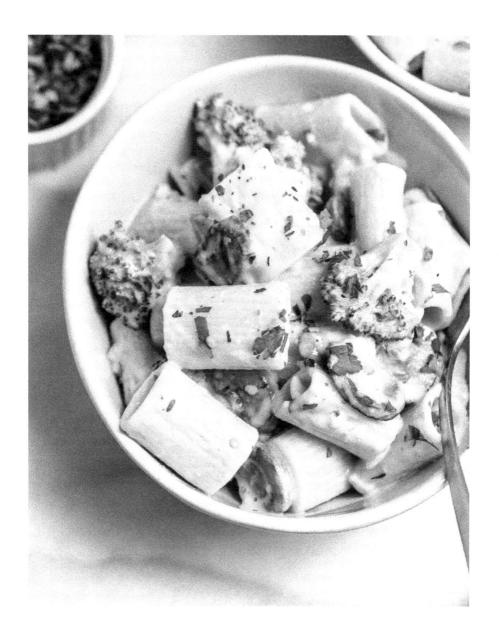

Preparation Time: 10 mins Servings: 2

Ingredients:

2   tsps. Minced garlic

2 c. Broccoli florets

Freshly ground black pepper

2 tbsps. Parmesan cheese

1/3 lb. Rigatoni noodles

2 tsps. Olive oil

Directions:

1.   Fill a pot three-quarters of the way full with water and bring it to a boil. Add the rigatoni and cook until it is firm, around twelve minutes. Drain it thoroughly.

2.   As the pasta cooks, bring an inch of water to a boil and put a steamer basket over the top. Add the broccoli and steam for ten minutes.

3.   In a bowl, mix together the pasta and broccoli. Toss with the cheese, oil, and garlic.

4.   Season to taste and serve.

Nutrition: Calories: 355, Fat:7 g, Carbs:63 g, Protein:14 g, Sugars:4 g, Sodium:600 mg

Vegan Rice Pudding

Preparation Time: 5 mins Servings: 8

Ingredients:

½ tsp. ground cinnamon

1 c. rinsed basmati

1/8 tsp. ground cardamom

¼ c. sugar

1/8 tsp. pure almond extract

1 quart vanilla nondairy milk

1 tsp. pure vanilla extract

Directions:

1.   Measure all of the ingredients into a saucepan and stir well to combine. Bring to a boil over medium- high heat.

2.   Once boiling, reduce heat to low and simmer, stirring very frequently, about 15–20 minutes.

3.   Remove from heat and cool. Serve sprinkled with additional ground cinnamon if desired.

Nutrition: Calories: 148, Fat:2 g, Carbs:26 g, Protein:4 g, Sugars:35 g, Sodium:150 mg

Cinnamon-Scented Quinoa

Preparation Time: 5 mins Servings: 4

Ingredients:

Chopped walnuts

1 ½ c. water Maple syrup

2 cinnamon sticks

1 c. quinoa

Directions:

1.   Add the quinoa to a bowl and wash it in several changes of water until the water is clear. When washing quinoa, rub grains and allow them to settle before you pour off the water.

2.   Use a large fine-mesh sieve to drain the quinoa. Prepare your pressure cooker with a trivet and steaming basket. Place the quinoa and the cinnamon sticks in the basket and pour the water.

3.   Close and lock the lid. Cook at high pressure for 6 minutes. When the cooking time is up, release the pressure using the quick release method.

4.   Fluff the quinoa with a fork and remove the cinnamon sticks. Divide the cooked quinoa among serving bowls and top with maple syrup and chopped walnuts.

Nutrition: Calories: 160, Fat:3 g, Carbs:28 g, Protein:6 g, Sugars:19 g, Sodium:40 mg

Green Vegetable Smoothie

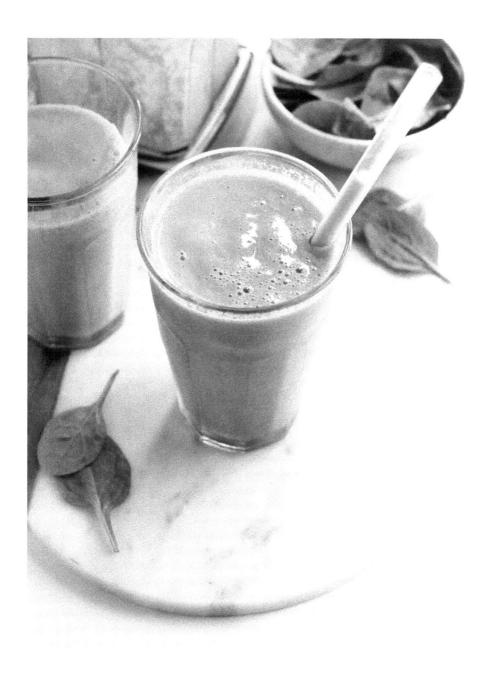

Preparation Time: 5 mins Servings: 4

Ingredients:

1 c. cold water

½ c. strawberries

2 oz. baby spinach 1 lemon juice

1 tbsp. fresh mint 1 banana

½ c. blueberries

Directions:

1. Put all the ingredients in a juicer or blender and puree.

Nutrition: Calories: 52, Fat:2 g, Carbs:12 g, Protein:1 g, Sugars:18 g, Sodium:36 mg

Garlic Lovers Hummus

Preparation Time: 2 mins Servings: 12

Ingredients:

3 tbsps. Freshly squeezed lemon juice

All-purpose salt-free seasoning

3 tbsps. Sesame tahini

4 garlic cloves

15 oz. no-salt-added garbanzo beans

2 tbsps. Olive oil

Directions:

1.   Drain garbanzo beans and rinse well.

2.   Place all the ingredients in a food processor and pulse until smooth.

3.   Serve immediately or cover and refrigerate until serving.

Nutrition: Calories: 103, Fat:5 g, Carbs:11 g, Protein:4 g, Sugars:2 g, Sodium:88 mg

Spinach and Kale Mix

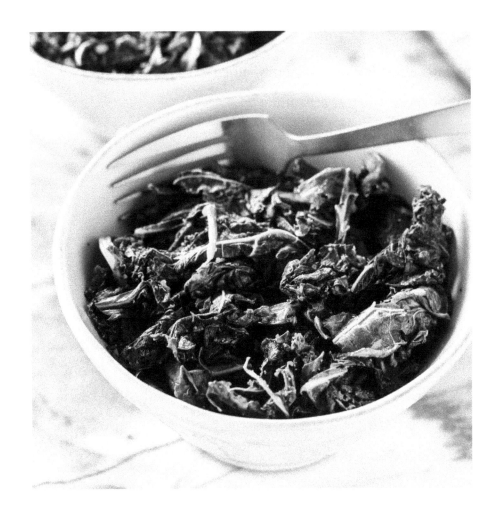

Preparation Time: 5 mins Servings: 4

Ingredients:

2 chopped shallots

1   c. no-salt-added and chopped canned tomatoes

2 c. baby spinach

2   minced garlic cloves

5 c. torn kale

1   tbsp. olive oil

Directions:

1.   Heat up a pan with the oil over medium-high heat, add the shallots, stir and sauté for 5 minutes.

2.   Add the spinach, kale and the other ingredients, toss, cook for 10 minutes more, divide between plates and serve.

Nutrition: Calories: 89, Fat:3.7 g, Carbs:12.4 g, Protein:3.6 g, Sugars:0 g, Sodium:50 mg

Apples and Cabbage Mix

Preparation Time: 5 mins Servings: 4

Ingredients:

2   cored and cubed green apples

2 tbsps. balsamic vinegar

½ tsp. caraway seeds

2 tbsps. olive oil

Black pepper

1 shredded red cabbage head

Directions:

1.   In a bowl, combine the cabbage with the apples and the other ingredients, toss and serve.

Nutrition: Calories: 165, Fat:7.4 g, Carbs:26 g, Protein:2.6 g, Sugars:2.6 g, Sodium:19 mg

Puréed Broccoli and Cauliflower

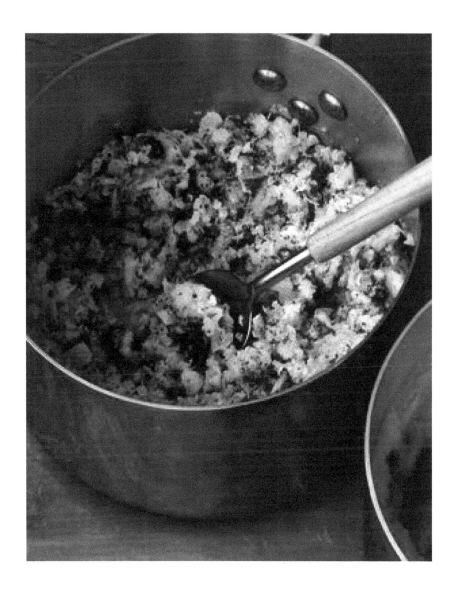

Preparation time: 10 minutes Cooking time: 15 minutes Servings: 5

Ingredients:

1   cauliflower head, separated into florets

1 broccoli head, separated into florets

Salt and ground black pepper, to taste

2   garlic cloves, peeled and minced 2

bacon slices, chopped

2 tablespoons butter

Directions:

1.   Heat up a pot with the butter over medium-high heat, add the garlic and bacon, stir, and cook for 3 minutes.

2.   Add the cauliflower and broccoli florets, stir, and cook for 2 minutes. Add the water to cover them, cover the pot, and simmer for 10 minutes.

3.   Add the salt and pepper, stir again, and blend soup using an immersion blender. Simmer for a couple minutes over medium heat, ladle into bowls, and serve.

Nutrition: Calories - 230, Fat - 3, Fiber - 3, Carbs - 6, Protein - 10

Broccoli Stew

Preparation time: 10 minutes Cooking time: 40 minutes Servings: 4

Ingredients:

1 broccoli head, separated into florets

2 teaspoons coriander seeds

A drizzle of olive oil

1 onion, peeled and chopped

Salt and ground black pepper, to taste

A pinch of red pepper, crushed

1 small ginger piece, peeled, and chopped

1 garlic clove, peeled and minced

28 ounces canned pureed tomatoes

Directions:

1.   Put water in a pot, add the salt, bring to a boil over medium-high heat, add the broccoli florets, steam them for 2 minutes, transfer them to a bowl filled with ice water, drain them, and leave aside.

2.   Heat up a pan over medium-high heat, add the coriander seeds, toast them for 4 minutes, transfer to a grinder, ground them, and set aside as well.

3.   Heat up a pot with the oil over medium heat, add the onions, salt, pepper, and red pepper, stir, and cook for 7 minutes.

4.   Add the ginger, garlic, and coriander seeds, stir, and cook for 3 minutes.

5.   Add the tomatoes, bring to a boil, and simmer for 10 minutes.

6.   Add the broccoli, stir and cook the stew for 12 minutes.

7.   Divide into bowls and serve.

Nutrition: Calories - 150, Fat - 4, Fiber - 2, Carbs - 5, Protein - 12

Bok Choy Soup

Preparation time: 10 minutes Cooking time: 15 minutes Servings: 4

Ingredients:

3 cups beef stock

1 onion, peeled and chopped

1 bunch bok choy, chopped 1½ cups mushrooms, chopped

Salt and ground black pepper, to taste

½ tablespoon red pepper flakes 3 tablespoons coconut aminos

3 tablespoons Parmesan cheese, grated 2 tablespoons Worcestershire sauce

2 bacon strips, chopped

Directions:

1.   Heat up a pot over medium-high heat, add the bacon, stir, cook until it until crispy, transfer to paper towels, and drain the grease.

2.   Heat up the pot again over medium heat, add the mushrooms and onions, stir, and cook for 5 minutes.

3.   Add the stock, bok choy, coconut aminos, salt, pepper, pepper flakes, and Worcestershire sauce, stir, cover, and cook until bok choy is tender.

4.   Ladle the soup into bowls, sprinkle Parmesan cheese, and bacon, and serve.

Nutrition: Calories - 100, Fat - 3, Fiber - 1, Carbs - 2, Protein - 6

Bok Choy Stir-fry

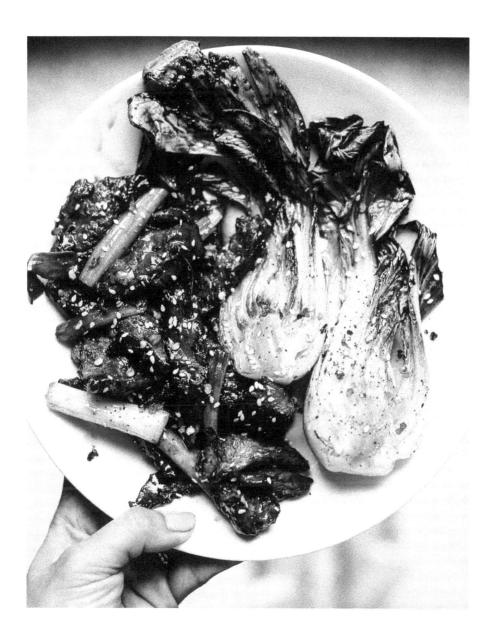

Preparation time: 10 minutes Cooking time: 7 minutes Servings: 2

Ingredients:

2 garlic cloves, peeled and minced

2 cup bok choy, chopped

2 bacon slices, chopped

Salt and ground black pepper, to taste

A drizzle of avocado oil

Directions:

1.   Heat up a pan with the oil over medium heat, add the bacon, stir, and brown until crispy, transfer to paper towels, and drain the grease.

2.   Return the pan to medium heat, add the garlic and bok choy, stir, and cook for 4 minutes.

3.   Add the salt, pepper, and return the bacon to the pan, stir, cook for 1 minute, divide on plates, and serve.

Nutrition: Calories - 50, Fat - 1, Fiber - 1, Carbs - 2, Protein - 2

Cream of Celery Soup

Preparation time: 10 minutes Cooking time: 40 minutes Servings: 4

Ingredients:

1 bunch celery, chopped

Salt and ground black pepper, to taste

3 bay leaves

½ garlic head, peeled, and chopped

2 onions, peeled and chopped

4 cups chicken stock

¾ cup heavy cream

2 tablespoons butter

Directions:

1.   Heat up a pot with the butter over medium-high heat, add the onions, salt, and pepper, stir, and cook for 5 minutes.

2.   Add the bay leaves, garlic, and celery, stir, and cook for 15 minutes.

3.   Add the stock, more salt and pepper, stir, cover the pot, reduce the heat, and simmer for 20 minutes.

4.   Add the cream, stir, and blend everything using an immersion blender.

5.   Ladle into soup bowls and serve.

Nutrition: Calories - 150, Fat - 3, Fiber - 1, Carbs - 2, Protein - 6

Celery Soup

Preparation time: 10 minutes Cooking time: 25 minutes Servings: 8

Ingredients:

26 ounces celery leaves, and stalks, chopped

1 tablespoon dried onion flakes

Salt and ground black pepper, to taste

3 teaspoons fenugreek powder

3 teaspoons vegetable stock powder

10 ounces sour cream

Directions:

1. Put the celery into a pot, add the water to cover, add the onion flakes, salt, pepper, stock powder, and fenugreek powder, stir, bring to a boil over medium heat, and simmer for 20 minutes.

2. Use an immersion blender to make the cream, add the sour cream, more salt and pepper, and blend again.

3. Heat up soup again over medium heat, ladle into bowls, and serve.

Nutrition: Calories - 140, Fat - 2, Fiber - 1, Carbs - 5, Protein - 10

Celery Stew

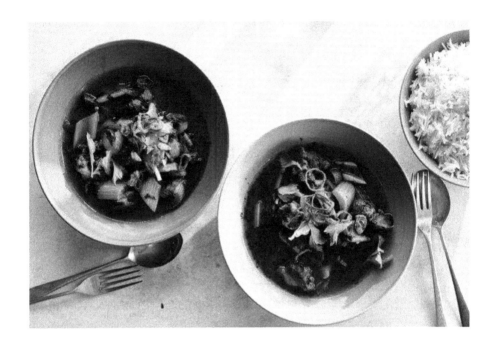

Preparation time: 10 minutes Cooking time: 30 minutes Servings: 6

Ingredients:

1 celery bunch, chopped

1 onion, peeled and chopped

1   bunch green onion, peeled and chopped

4 garlic cloves, peeled and minced

Salt and ground black pepper, to taste

1 fresh parsley bunch, chopped

2   fresh mint bunches, chopped

3   dried Persian lemons, pricked with a fork

 2 cups water

2 teaspoons chicken bouillon 4 tablespoons olive oil

Directions:

1.   Heat up a pot with the oil over medium-high heat, add the onion, green onions, and garlic, stir, and cook for 6 minutes.

2.   Add the celery, Persian lemons, chicken bouillon, salt, pepper, and water, stir, cover pot, and simmer on medium heat for 20 minutes.

3.   Add the parsley and mint, stir, and cook for 10 minutes.

4.   Divide into bowls and serve.

Nutrition: Calories - 170, Fat - 7, Fiber - 4, Carbs - 6, Protein - 10

Spinach Soup

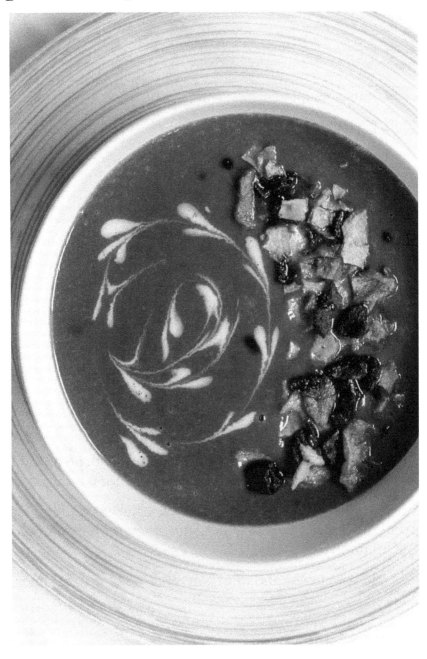

Preparation time: 10 minutes Cooking time: 15 minutes Servings: 8

Ingredients:

2 tablespoons butter

20 ounces spinach, chopped

1 teaspoon garlic, minced

Salt and ground black pepper, to taste

45 ounces chicken stock

½ teaspoon ground nutmeg

2 cups heavy cream

1   onion, peeled and chopped

Directions:

1.   Heat up a pot with the butter over medium heat, add the onion, stir, and cook for 4 minutes.

2.   Add the garlic, stir, and cook for 1 minute.

3.   Add the spinach and stock, stir, and cook for 5 minutes.

4.   Blend soup with an immersion blender, and heat up the soup again.

5.   Add the salt, pepper, nutmeg, and cream, stir, and cook for 5 minutes.

6.   Ladle into bowls and serve.

Nutrition: Calories - 245, Fat - 24, Fiber - 3, Carbs - 4, Protein - 6

Sautéed Mustard Greens

Preparation time: 5 minutes Cooking time: 15 minutes

Servings: 4

Ingredients:

2   garlic cloves, peeled and minced

1 pound mustard greens, torn

1 tablespoon olive oil

½ cup onion, sliced

Salt and ground black pepper, to taste

3 tablespoons vegetable stock

¼ teaspoon dark sesame oil

Directions:

1.   Heat up a pan with the oil over medium heat, add the onions, stir, and brown them for 10 minutes.

2.   Add the garlic, stir, and cook for 1 minute.

3.   Add the stock, greens, salt, and pepper, stir, and cook for 5 minutes.

4.   Add more salt and pepper, and sesame oil, toss to coat, divide on plates, and serve.

Nutrition: Calories - 120, Fat - 3, Fiber - 1, Carbs - 3, Protein - 6

Collard Greens and Poached Eggs

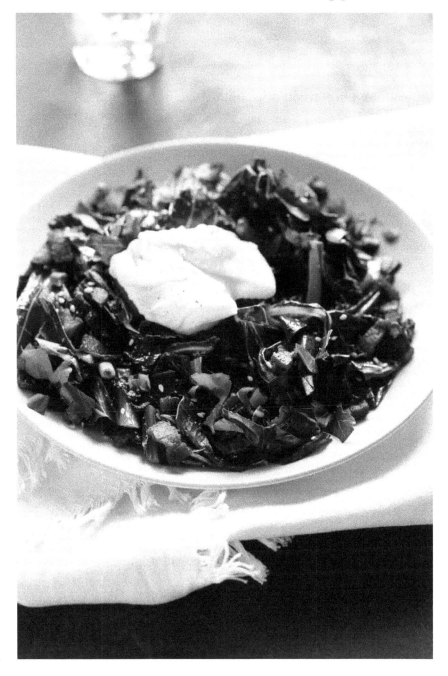

Preparation time: 10 minutes Cooking time: 15 minutes Servings: 6

Ingredients:

1 tablespoon chipotle in adobo, mashed

6 eggs

3 tablespoons butter

1   onion, peeled and chopped

2   garlic cloves, peeled and minced

6 bacon slices, chopped

3   bunches collard greens, chopped

½ cup chicken stock

Salt and ground black pepper, to taste

1 tablespoon lime juice

Cheddar cheese, grated, for serving

Directions:

1.   Heat up a pan over medium-high heat, add the bacon, cook until crispy, transfer to paper towels, drain grease, and leave aside.

2.   Heat up the pan again over medium heat, add the garlic and onion, stir, and cook for 2 minutes.

3.   Return the bacon to the pan, stir, and cook for 3 minutes.

4.   Add the chipotle in adobo paste, collard greens, salt, and pepper, stir, and cook for 10 minutes.

5.   Add the stock and lime juice, and stir.

6.   Make 6 holes in collard greens mixture, divide butter in them, crack an egg in each hole, cover the pan, and cook until eggs are done.

7.   Divide this on plates and serve with cheddar cheese sprinkled on top.

Nutrition: Calories - 245, Fat - 20, Fiber - 1, Carbs - 5, Protein - 12

Collard Greens Soup

Preparation time: 10 minutes Cooking time: 40 minutes Servings: 12

Ingredients:

1   teaspoon chili powder

1 tablespoon avocado oil

2   teaspoons smoked paprika

1 teaspoon cumin

1 onion, peeled and chopped A pinch of red pepper flakes

10 cups water

3 celery stalks, chopped

3 carrots, peeled and chopped

15 ounces canned diced tomatoes

2 tablespoons tamari sauce

6 ounces canned tomato paste

2 tablespoons lemon juice

Salt and ground black pepper, to taste

6 cups collard greens, stems discarded

1 tablespoon swerve

1 teaspoon dried garlic

1   tablespoon herb seasoning

Directions:

1.   Heat up a pot with the oil over medium-high heat, add the cumin, pepper flakes, paprika, and chili powder, and stir well.

2.   Add the celery, onion, and carrots, stir, and cook for 10 minutes.

3.   Add the tamari sauce, tomatoes, tomato paste, water, lemon juice, salt, pepper, herb seasoning, swerve, garlic granules, and collard greens, stir, bring to a boil, cover, and cook for 30 minutes.

4.   Stir again, ladle into bowls, and serve.

Nutrition: Calories - 150, Fat - 3, Fiber - 2, Carbs - 4, Protein – 8

Spring Greens Soup

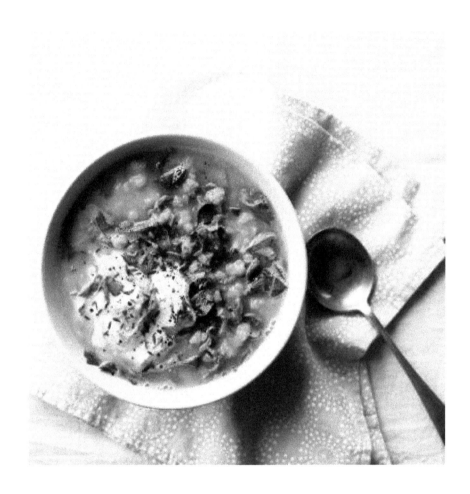

Preparation time: 10 minutes Cooking time: 30 minutes Servings: 4

Ingredients:

2   cups mustard greens, chopped

2 cups collard greens, chopped

3 quarts vegetable stock

1   onion, peeled and chopped

Salt and ground black pepper, to taste

2 tablespoons coconut aminos

2   teaspoons fresh ginger, grated

Directions:

1.   Put the stock into a pot, and bring to a simmer over medium-high heat.

2.   Add the mustard, collard greens, onion, salt, pepper, coconut aminos, and ginger, stir, cover the pot, and cook for 30 minutes.

3.   Blend the soup using an immersion blender, add more salt, and pepper, heat up over medium heat, ladle into soup bowls, and serve.

Nutrition: Calories - 140, Fat - 2, Fiber - 1, Carbs - 3, Protein - 7

Mustard Greens and Spinach Soup

Preparation time: 10 minutes Cooking time: 15 minutes Servings: 6

Ingredients:

½ teaspoon fenugreek seeds

1 teaspoon cumin seeds

1 tablespoon avocado oil

1 teaspoon coriander seeds

1 cup onion, chopped

1 tablespoon garlic, minced

1 tablespoon fresh ginger, grated

½ teaspoon turmeric

5 cups mustard greens, chopped

3 cups coconut milk

1 tablespoon jalapeño, chopped

5 cups spinach, torn

Salt and ground black pepper, to taste

2 teaspoons butter

½ teaspoon paprika

Directions:

1.   Heat up a pot with the oil over medium-high heat, add the coriander, fenugreek, and cumin seeds, stir, and brown them for 2 minutes.

2.   Add the onions, stir, and cook for 3 minutes. Add the half of the garlic, jalapeños, ginger, and turmeric, stir, and cook for 3 minutes.

3.   Add the mustard greens, and spinach, stir, and sauté everything for 10 minutes.

4.   Add the milk, salt, and pepper, and blend the soup using an immersion blender.

5.   Heat up a pan with the butter over medium heat, add the garlic, and paprika, stir well, and take off the heat.

6.   Heat up the soup over medium heat, ladle into soup bowls, drizzle with butter and sprinkle with paprika all over, and serve.

Nutrition: Calories - 143, Fat - 6, Fiber - 3, Carbs - 7, Protein - 7

Roasted Asparagus

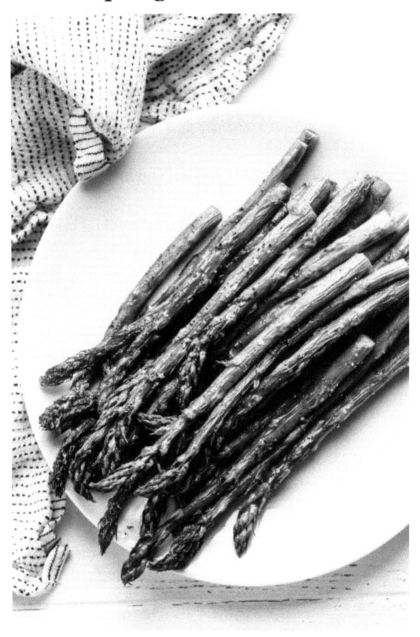

Preparation time: 10 minutes Cooking time: 10 minutes Servings: 3

Ingredients:

1 asparagus bunch, trimmed

3 teaspoons avocado oil

A splash of lemon juice

Salt and ground black pepper, to taste

1 tablespoon fresh oregano, chopped

Directions:

1.   Spread the asparagus spears on a lined baking sheet, season with salt, and pepper, drizzle with oil and lemon juice, sprinkle with oregano, and toss to coat well.

2.   Place in an oven at 425°F, and bake for 10 minutes.

3.   Divide on plates and serve.

Nutrition: Calories - 130, Fat - 1, Fiber - 1, Carbs - 2, Protein - 3

Asparagus and Browned Butter

Preparation time: 10 minutes Cooking time: 15 minutes Servings: 4

Ingredients:

5 ounces butter

1 tablespoon avocado oil

1½ pounds asparagus, trimmed

1½ tablespoons lemon juice

A pinch of cayenne pepper

8 tablespoons sour cream

Salt and ground black pepper, to taste

3 ounces Parmesan cheese, grated

4 eggs

Directions:

1.   Heat up a pan with 2 ounces butter over medium-high heat, add the eggs, some salt and pepper, stir, and scramble them.

2.   Transfer the eggs to a blender, add the Parmesan cheese, sour cream, salt, pepper, and cayenne pepper, and blend everything well.

3.   Heat up a pan with the oil over medium-high heat, add the asparagus, salt, and pepper, roast for a few minutes, transfer to a plate, and set aside.

4.   Heat up the pan again with the rest of the butter over medium-high heat, stir until brown, take off the heat, add the lemon juice, and stir well.

5.   Heat up the butter again, return the asparagus to the pan, toss to coat, heat up well, and divide on plates.

6.   Add the blended eggs on top and serve.

Nutrition: Calories - 160, Fat - 7, Fiber - 2, Carbs - 6, Protein - 10

Asparagus Frittata

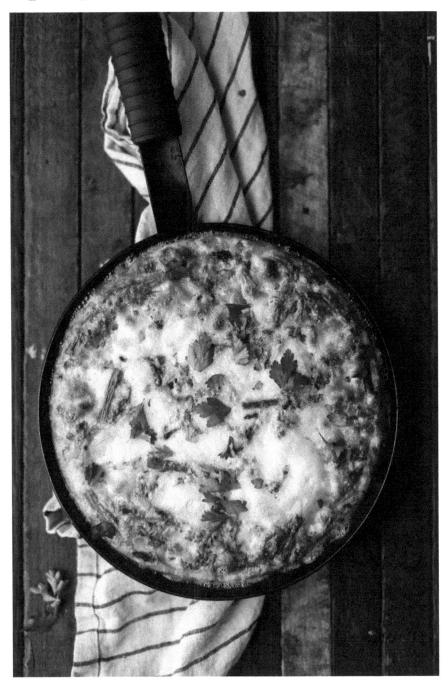

Preparation time: 10 minutes Cooking time: 15 minutes Servings: 4

Ingredients:

¼ cup onion, chopped

A drizzle of olive oil

1 pound asparagus spears, cut into 1-inch pieces

Salt and ground black pepper, to taste

4 eggs, whisked

1 cup cheddar cheese, grated

Directions:

1.   Heat up a pan with the oil over medium-high heat, add the onions, stir, and cook for 3 minutes.

2.   Add the asparagus, stir, and cook for 6 minutes.

3.   Add the eggs, stir, and cook for 3 minutes.

4.   Add the salt and pepper, sprinkle with the cheese, place in an oven, and broil for 3 minutes.

5.   Divide the frittata on plates and serve.

Nutrition: Calories - 200, Fat - 12, Fiber - 2, Carbs - 5, Protein - 14

Creamy Asparagus

Preparation time: 10 minutes Cooking time: 15 minutes Servings: 3

Ingredients:

10 ounces asparagus spears, cut into medium-sized pieces, and steamed

Salt and ground black pepper, to taste

2 tablespoons

Parmesan cheese, grated

⅓ cup Monterey jack cheese, shredded

2 tablespoons mustard

2   ounces cream cheese

⅓ cup heavy cream

3   tablespoons bacon, cooked and crumbled

Directions:

1.   Heat up a pan with the mustard, heavy cream, and cream cheese over medium heat and stir well.

2.   Add the Monterey Jack cheese, and Parmesan cheese, stir, and cook until it melts.

3.   Add the half of the bacon, and the asparagus, stir, and cook for 3 minutes.

4.   Add the rest of the bacon, plus salt and pepper, stir, cook for 5 minutes, divide on plates, and serve.

Nutrition: Calories - 256, Fat - 23, Fiber - 2, Carbs - 5, Protein - 13

Alfalfa Sprouts Salad

Preparation time: 10 minutes Cooking time: 0 minutes Servings: 4

Ingredients:

1   green apple, cored, and julienned

1½ teaspoons dark sesame oil

4 cups alfalfa sprouts

Salt and ground black pepper, to taste

1½ teaspoons grape seed oil

¼ cup coconut milk yogurt

4 nasturtium leaves

Directions:

1.   In a salad bowl, mix the sprouts with apple and nasturtium.

2.   Add the salt, pepper, sesame oil, grape seed oil, and coconut yogurt, toss to coat, and divide on plates, and serve.

Nutrition: Calories - 100, Fat - 3, Fiber - 1, Carbs - 2, Protein - 6

Roasted Radishes

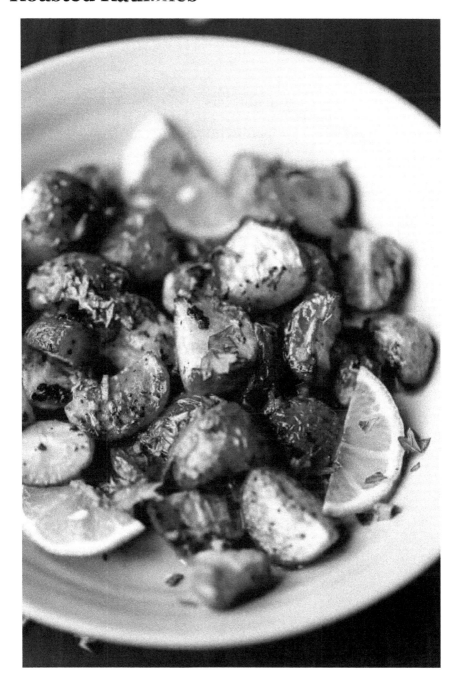

Preparation time: 10 minutes Cooking time: 35 minutes Servings: 2

Ingredients:

2 cups radishes, cut in quarters

Salt and ground black pepper, to taste

2 tablespoons butter, melted

1 tablespoon fresh chives, chopped

1 tablespoon lemon zest

Directions:

1. Spread the radishes on a lined baking sheet.

2. Add the salt, pepper, chives, lemon zest, and butter, toss to coat, and bake in the oven at 375°F for 35 minutes.

3. Divide on plates and serve.

Nutrition: Calories - 122, Fat - 12, Fiber - 1, Carbs - 3, Protein - 14

Crispy Radishes

Preparation time: 10 minutes Cooking time: 20 minutes Servings: 4

Ingredients:

Vegetable oil cooking spray

15 radishes, sliced

Salt and ground black pepper, to taste

1 tablespoon fresh chives, chopped

Directions:

1.   Arrange the radish slices on a lined baking sheet and spray them with cooking oil.

2.   Season with salt and pepper, sprinkle with the chives, place in an oven at 375°F, and bake for 10 minutes.

3.   Flip them and bake for 10 minutes.

4.   Serve cold.

Nutrition: Calories - 30, Fat - 1, Fiber - 0. 4, Carbs - 1, Protein - 0. 1

Creamy Radishes

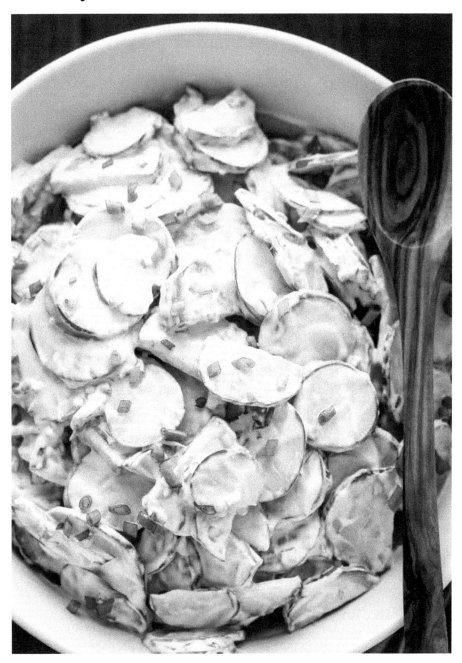

Preparation time: 10 minutes Cooking time: 25 minutes Servings: 1

Ingredients:

7 ounces radishes, cut in half

2 tablespoons sour cream

2 bacon slices

1   tablespoon green onion, peeled and chopped

1 tablespoon cheddar cheese, grated

Hot sauce, to taste

Salt and ground black pepper, to taste

Directions:

1.   Put the radishes into a pot, add the water to cover, bring to a boil over medium heat, cook them for 10 minutes, and drain.

2.   Heat up a pan over medium-high heat, add the bacon, cook until crispy, transfer to paper towels, drain the grease, crumble, and leave aside.

3.   Return the pan to medium heat, add the radishes, stir, and sauté them for 7 minutes.

4.   Add the onion, salt, pepper, hot sauce, and sour cream, stir, and cook for 7 minutes.

5.   Transfer to a plate, top with crumbled bacon and cheddar cheese, and serve.

Nutrition: Calories - 340, Fat - 23, Fiber - 3, Carbs - 6, Protein - 15

Radish Soup

Preparation time: 10 minutes Cooking time: 20 minutes Servings: 4

Ingredients:

2   bunches radishes, cut in quarters

Salt and ground black pepper, to taste

 6 cups chicken stock

2 stalks celery, chopped

 3 tablespoons coconut oil

6 garlic cloves, peeled and minced

1 onion, peeled and chopped

Directions:

1.   Heat up a pot with the oil over medium heat, add the onion, celery, and garlic, stir, and cook for 5 minutes.

2.   Add the radishes, stock, salt, and pepper, stir, bring to a boil, cover, and simmer for 15 minutes.

3.   Divide into soup bowls and serve.

Nutrition: Calories - 120, Fat - 2, Fiber - 1, Carbs - 3, Protein - 10

Avocado Salad

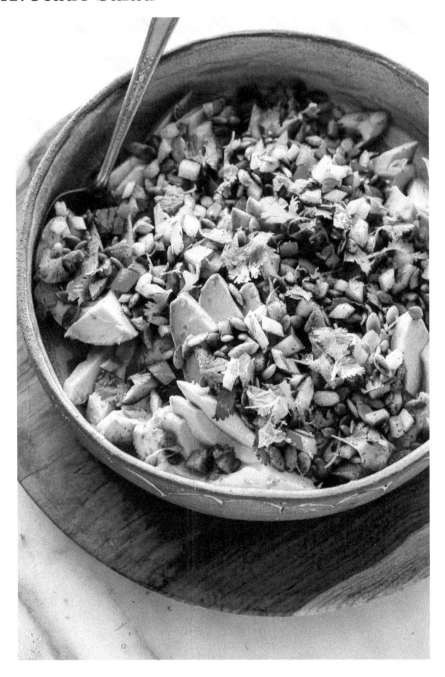

Preparation time: 10 minutes Cooking time: 0 minutes Servings: 4

Ingredients:

2 avocados, pitted, and mashed

Salt and ground black pepper, to taste

¼ teaspoon lemon stevia

1 tablespoon white vinegar

14 ounces coleslaw mix

Juice from 2 limes

¼ cup onion, chopped

¼ cup fresh cilantro, chopped

2 tablespoons olive oil

Directions:

1.   Put the coleslaw mixture in a salad bowl.

2.   Add the avocado mash and onions, and toss to coat.

3.   In a bowl, mix the lime juice with salt, pepper, oil, vinegar, and stevia, and stir well.

4.   Add this to salad, toss to coat, sprinkle cilantro, and serve.

Nutrition: Calories - 100, Fat - 10, Fiber - 2, Carbs - 5, Protein - 8

Avocado and Egg Salad

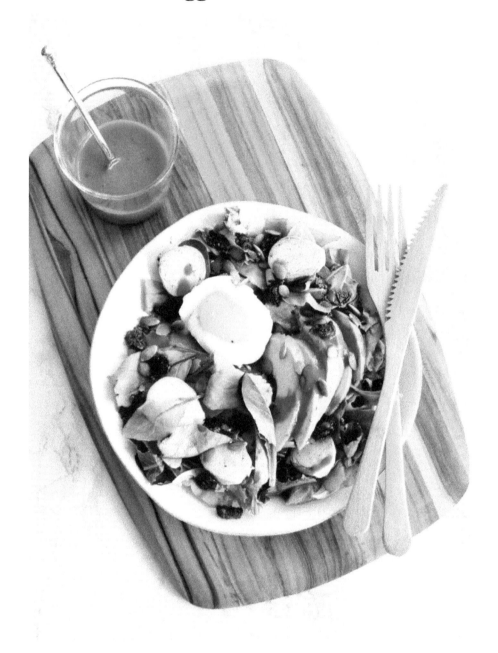

Preparation time: 10 minutes Cooking time: 7 minutes

Servings: 4

Ingredients:

4 cups mixed lettuce leaves, torn

4 eggs

1   avocado, pitted, and sliced

¼ cup mayonnaise

2 teaspoons mustard

2   garlic cloves, peeled and minced

1 tablespoon fresh chives, chopped

Salt and ground black pepper, to taste

Directions:

1.   Put water in a pot, add some salt, add the eggs, bring to a boil over medium-high heat, boil for 7 minutes, drain, cool, peel, and chop them. In a salad bowl, mix the lettuce with eggs, and avocado.

2.   Add the chives and garlic, some salt, and pepper, and toss to coat.

3.   In a bowl, mix the mustard with mayonnaise, salt, and pepper, and stir well.

4.   Add this to the salad, toss well, and serve.

Nutrition: Calories - 234, Fat - 12, Fiber - 4, Carbs - 7, Protein - 12

Avocado and Cucumber Salad

Preparation time: 10 minutes Cooking time: 0 minutes Servings: 4

Ingredients:

1   onion, peeled and sliced

1 cucumber, sliced

2   avocados, pitted, peeled, and chopped

1 pound cherry tomatoes, halved

2 tablespoons olive oil

¼ cup fresh cilantro, chopped

2 tablespoons lemon juice

Salt and ground black pepper, to taste

Directions:

1.   In a large salad bowl, mix the tomatoes with the cucumber, onion, and avocado, and stir.

2.   Add the oil, salt, pepper, and lemon juice, and toss to coat well.

3.   Serve cold with cilantro on top.

Nutrition: Calories - 140, Fat - 4, Fiber - 2, Carbs - 4, Protein - 5

Arugula Salad

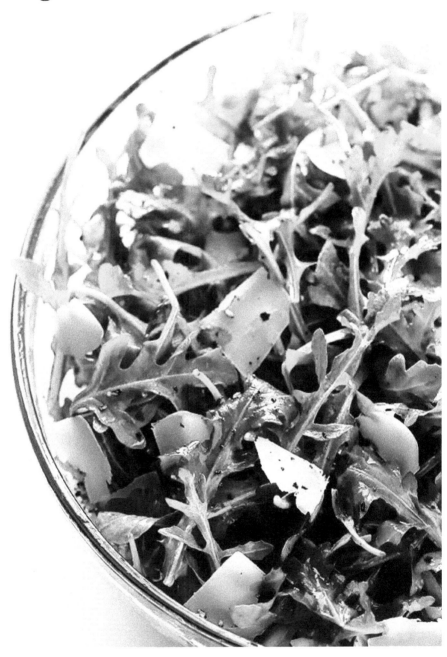

Preparation time: 10 minutes Cooking time: 0 minutes Servings: 4

Ingredients:

1 white onion, peeled and chopped

1 tablespoon vinegar

1 cup hot water

1   bunch baby arugula

¼ cup walnuts, chopped

2   tablespoons fresh cilantro, chopped

2 garlic cloves, peeled and minced

2 tablespoons olive oil

Salt and ground black pepper, to taste

1 tablespoon lemon juice

Directions:

1.   In a bowl, mix the water with vinegar, add the onion, set aside for 5 minutes, and drain well.

2.   In a salad bowl, mix the arugula with the walnuts and onion, and stir.

3.   Add the garlic, salt, pepper, lemon juice, cilantro, and oil, toss well, and serve.

Nutrition: Calories - 200, Fat - 2, Fiber - 1, Carbs - 5, Protein - 7

Arugula Soup

Preparation time: 10 minutes Cooking time: 13 minutes Servings: 6

Ingredients:

1   onion, peeled and chopped

1 tablespoon olive oil

2   garlic cloves, peeled and minced

½ cup coconut milk

10 ounces baby arugula

2 tablespoons fresh mint, chopped, and

2 tablespoons fresh tarragon, chopped

2 tablespoons fresh parsley, chopped

2 tablespoons fresh chives, chopped

4 tablespoons coconut milk yogurt

6 cups chicken stock

Salt and ground black pepper, to taste

Directions:

1.   Heat up a pot with the oil over medium-high heat, add the onion and garlic, stir, and cook for 5 minutes.

2.   Add the stock, and milk, stir, and bring to a simmer.

3.   Add the arugula, tarragon, parsley, and mint, stir, and cook for 6 minutes.

4.   Add the coconut yogurt, salt, pepper, and chives, stir, cook for 2 minutes, divide into soup bowls, and serve.

Nutrition: Calories - 200, Fat - 4, Fiber - 2, Carbs - 6, Protein - 10

Arugula and Broccoli Soup

Preparation time: 10 minutes Cooking time: 20 minutes Servings: 4

Ingredients:

1 onion, peeled and chopped

1 tablespoon olive oil

1 garlic clove, peeled and minced

1 broccoli head, separated into florets

Salt and ground black pepper, to taste

2, and ½ cups vegetable stock

1 teaspoon cumin

Juice of ½ lemon

1 cup arugula leaves

Directions:

1.   Heat up a pot with the oil over medium-high heat, add the onions, stir, and cook for 4 minutes.

2.   Add the garlic, stir, and cook for 1 minute.

3.   Add the broccoli, cumin, salt, and pepper, stir, and cook for 4 minutes.

4.   Add the stock, stir, and cook for 8 minutes.

5.   Blend the soup using an immersion blender, add half of the arugula, and blend again.

6.   Add the rest of the arugula, stir, and heat up the soup again.

7.   Add the lemon juice, stir, ladle into soup bowls, and serve.

Nutrition: Calories - 150, Fat - 3, Fiber - 1, Carbs - 3, Protein - 7

Zucchini Cream

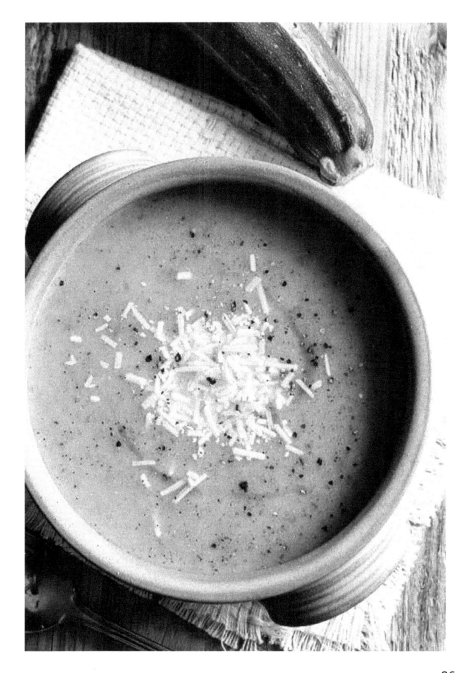

Preparation time: 10 minutes Cooking time: 25 minutes Servings: 8

Ingredients:

6 zucchini, cut in half and sliced

Salt and ground black pepper, to taste

1 tablespoon butter

28 ounces vegetable stock

1 teaspoon dried oregano

½ cup onion, chopped

3 garlic cloves, peeled and minced

2 ounces Parmesan cheese, grated

¾ cup heavy cream

Directions:

1.   Heat up a pot with the butter over medium-high heat, add the onion, stir, and cook for 4 minutes.

2.   Add the garlic, stir, and cook for 2 minutes.

3.   Add the zucchini, stir, and cook for 3 minutes.

4.   Add the stock, stir, bring to a boil, and simmer over medium heat for 15 minutes.

5.   Add the oregano, salt, and pepper, stir, take off the heat, and blend using an immersion blender.

6.   Heat the soup again, add the heavy cream, stir, and bring to a simmer.

7. Add the Parmesan cheese, stir, take off the heat, ladle into bowls, and serve.

Nutrition: Calories - 160, Fat - 4, Fiber - 2, Carbs - 4, Protein - 8

Swiss Chard Salad

Preparation time: 10 minutes Cooking time: 20 minutes Servings: 4

Ingredients:

1 bunch Swiss chard, cut into strips

2 tablespoons avocado oil

1 onion, peeled and chopped

A pinch of red pepper flakes

¼ cup pine nuts, toasted

¼ cup raisins

1 tablespoon balsamic vinegar

Salt and ground black pepper, to taste

Directions:

1.   Heat up a pan with the oil over medium heat, add the chard and onions, stir, and cook for 5 minutes.

2.   Add the salt, pepper, and pepper flakes, stir, and cook for 3 minutes.

3.   Put the raisins in a bowl, add the water to cover them, heat them up in a microwave for 1 minute, set aside for 5 minutes, and drain them well.

4.   Add the raisins, and pine nuts to the pan with the vinegar, stir, cook for 3 minutes, divide on plates, and serve.

Nutrition: Calories - 120, Fat - 2, Fiber - 1, Carbs - 4, Protein - 8

Green Salad

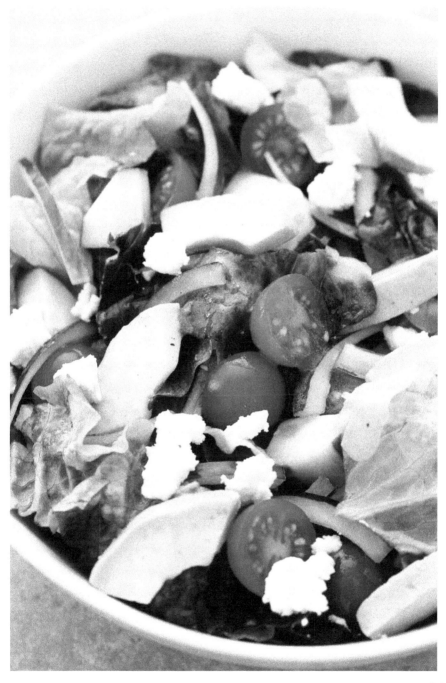

Preparation time: 10 minutes Cooking time: 0 minutes Servings: 4

Ingredients:

24 green grapes, halved

1 bunch Swiss chard, chopped

1 avocado, pitted, peeled, and cubed

Salt and ground black pepper, to taste

2 tablespoons avocado oil

1 tablespoon mustard 7 sage leaves, chopped

1 garlic clove, peeled and minced

Directions:

1. In a salad bowl, mix the Swiss chard with the grapes and avocado cubes.

2. In a bowl, mix the mustard with the oil, sage, garlic, salt, and pepper, and whisk.

3. Add this to the salad, toss to coat well, and serve.

Nutrition: Calories - 120, Fat - 2, Fiber - 1, Carbs - 4, Protein - 5

Catalan-style Greens

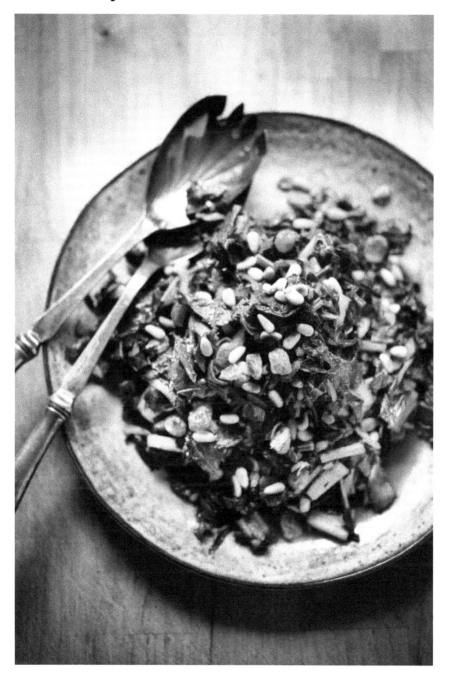

Preparation time: 10 minutes Cooking time: 15 minutes Servings: 4

Ingredients:

1 apple, cored and chopped

1 onion, peeled and sliced

3   tablespoons avocado oil

¼ cup raisins

6 garlic cloves, peeled and chopped

¼ cup pine nuts, toasted

¼ cup balsamic vinegar

2½ cups Swiss chard

2½ cups spinach, and

Salt and ground black pepper, to taste

A pinch of nutmeg

Directions:

1.   Heat up a pan with the oil over medium-high heat, add the onion, stir, and cook for 3 minutes.

2.   Add the apple, stir, and cook for 4 minutes.

3.   Add the garlic, stir, and cook for 1 minute.

4.   Add the raisins, vinegar, spinach, and chard, stir, and cook for 5 minutes.

5.   Add the nutmeg, salt, and pepper, stir, cook for a few seconds, divide on plates, and serve.

Nutrition: Calories - 120, Fat - 1, Fiber - 2, Carbs - 3, Protein - 6

Swiss Chard and Chicken Soup

Preparation time: 10 minutes Cooking time: 35 minutes Servings: 12

Ingredients:

4 cups Swiss chard, chopped

4 cups chicken breast, cooked, and shredded

2 cups water

1 cup mushrooms, sliced

1 tablespoon garlic, minced

1   tablespoon coconut oil, melted

¼ cup onion, peeled and chopped

8 cups chicken stock

2   cups yellow squash, chopped

1 cup green beans, cut into medium-sized pieces

2 tablespoons vinegar

¼ cup fresh basil, chopped

Salt and ground black pepper, to taste

4 bacon slices, chopped

¼ cup sundried tomatoes, cored and chopped

Directions:

1.   Heat up a pot with the oil over medium-high heat, add the bacon, stir, and cook for 2 minutes.

2.   Add the tomatoes, garlic, onions, and mushrooms, stir, and cook for 5 minutes.

3.   Add the water, stock, and chicken, stir, and cook for 15 minutes.

4.   Add the Swiss chard, green beans, squash, salt, and pepper, stir, and cook for 10 minutes.

5.   Add the vinegar, basil, salt, and pepper, stir, ladle into soup bowls, and serve.

Nutrition: Calories - 140, Fat - 4, Fiber - 2, Carbs - 4, Protein - 18

Roasted Tomato

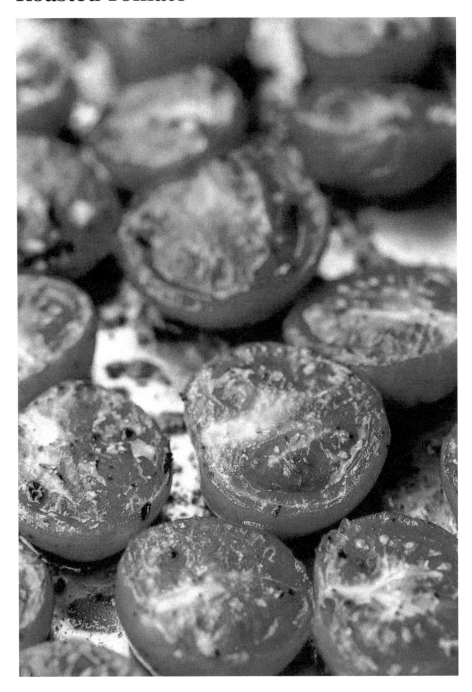

Cream Preparation time: 10 minutes Cooking time: 1 hour

Servings: 8

Ingredients:

1 jalapeño pepper, chopped

4 garlic cloves, peeled and minced

2 pounds cherry tomatoes, cut in half

1 onion, peeled and cut into wedges

Salt and ground black pepper, to taste

¼ cup olive oil

½ teaspoon dried oregano

4 cups chicken stock

¼ cup fresh basil, chopped

½ cup Parmesan cheese, grated

Directions:

1.   Spread the tomatoes, and onion in a baking dish.

2.   Add the garlic and chili pepper, season with salt, pepper, and oregano, and drizzle the oil.

3.   Toss to coat and bake in the oven at 425°F for 30 minutes.

4.   Take the tomato mixture out of the oven, transfer to a pot, add the stock, and heat everything up over medium-high heat.

5.   Bring to a boil, cover the pot, reduce heat, and simmer for 20 minutes.

6.   Blend using an immersion blender, add the salt and pepper to taste, and basil, stir, and ladle into soup bowls. Sprinkle with Parmesan cheese on top and serve.

Nutrition: Calories - 140, Fat - 2, Fiber - 2, Carbs - 5, Protein - 8

Eggplant Soup

Preparation time: 10 minutes Cooking time: 50 minutes Servings: 4

Ingredients:

4 tomatoes

1 teaspoon garlic, minced

¼ onion, peeled and chopped

Salt and ground black pepper, to taste

2 cups chicken stock

1   bay leaf

½ cup heavy cream

2   tablespoons fresh basil, chopped

4 tablespoons Parmesan cheese, grated

1 tablespoon olive oil

1 eggplant, chopped

Directions:

1.   Spread the eggplant pieces on a baking sheet, mix with oil, onion, garlic, salt, and pepper, place in an oven at 400°F, and bake for 15 minutes.

2.   Put water in a pot, bring to a boil over medium heat, add the tomatoes, steam them for 1 minute, peel them, and chop.

3.   Take the eggplant mixture out of the oven, and transfer to a pot.

4. Add the tomatoes, stock, bay leaf, salt, and pepper, stir, bring to a boil, and simmer for 30 minutes.

5. Add the heavy cream, basil, and Parmesan cheese, stir, ladle into soup bowls, and serve.

Nutrition: Calories - 180, Fat - 2, Fiber - 3, Carbs - 5, Protein - 10

Eggplant Stew

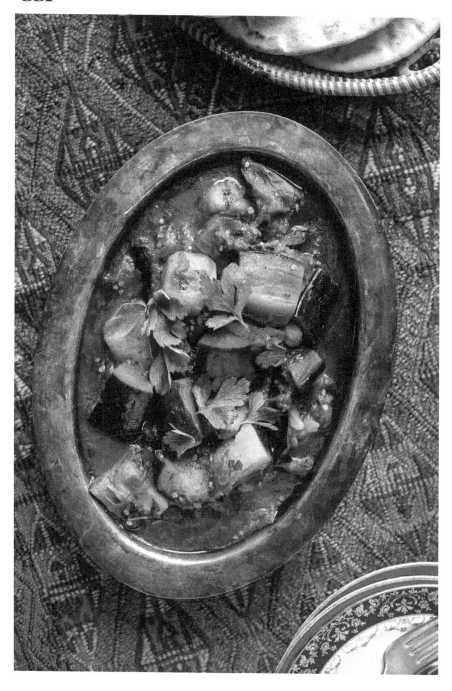

Preparation time: 10 minutes Cooking time: 30 minutes

Servings: 4

Ingredients:

1   onion, peeled and chopped

2   garlic cloves, peeled and chopped

1 bunch fresh parsley, chopped

Salt and ground black pepper, to taste

1 teaspoon dried oregano

2 eggplants, cut into medium-sized chunks

2 tablespoons olive oil

2 tablespoons capers, chopped

12 green olives, pitted and sliced

5 tomatoes, cored and chopped

3 tablespoons herb vinegar

Directions:

1.   Heat up a pot with the oil over medium heat, add the eggplant, oregano, salt, and pepper, stir, and cook for 5 minutes.

2.   Add the garlic, onion, and parsley, stir, and cook for 4 minutes.

3.   Add the capers, olives, vinegar, and tomatoes, stir, and cook for 15 minutes.

4. Add more salt and pepper, if needed, stir, divide into bowls, and serve.

Nutrition: Calories - 200, Fat - 13, Fiber - 3, Carbs - 5, Protein - 7

Roasted Bell Peppers Soup

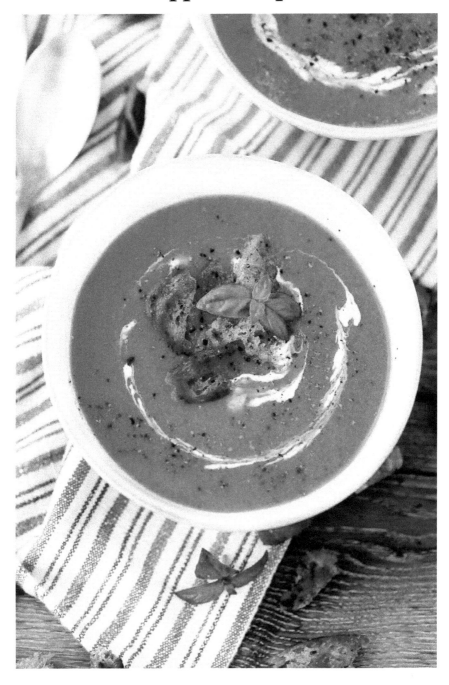

Preparation time: 10 minutes Cooking time: 15 minutes Servings: 6

Ingredients:

12 ounces roasted bell peppers, seeded and chopped

2 tablespoons olive oil

2 garlic cloves, peeled and minced

29 ounces canned chicken stock

Salt and ground black pepper, to taste

7 ounces water

⅔ cup heavy cream

1 onion, peeled and chopped

¼ cup Parmesan cheese, grated

2 celery stalks, chopped

Directions:

1.   Heat up a pot with the oil over medium heat, add the onion, garlic, celery, and some salt, and pepper, stir, and cook for 8 minutes.

2.   Add the bell peppers, water, and stock, stir, bring to a boil, cover, reduce the heat, and simmer for 5 minutes.

3.   Use an immersion blender to puree the soup, then add more salt, pepper, and cream, stir, bring to a boil, and take off the heat.

4.   Ladle into bowls, sprinkle Parmesan cheese, and serve.

Nutrition: Calories - 176, Fat - 13, Fiber - 1, Carbs - 4, Protein – 6

Lightning Source UK Ltd.
Milton Keynes UK
UKHW021016030521
383041UK00001B/58

9 781801 458153